# COPYRIGHT AND DISCLAIMER

I0122105

Expert Consultants: Saleema Noon & Tara Johnson
Research: Yasaman Madanikia
Cover Design: New Media Graphix
ISBN: 978-0-9918904-5-3

© GoTo Educational Technology Inc. 2013

# PREFACE

Why is teaching preschool children about sexual health so important? Well, for one thing, it's well documented that teaching children about sex and sexuality early helps prevent sexual abuse. But it's more than that, sexuality goes way beyond sexual intercourse and reproduction. Sexuality influences how we view ourselves and our bodies, how we interact with people, how we fit into our world and how we express ourselves as individuals. It's a dynamic process and will change as we learn and grow. Think of it as a journey, not a destination! As parents or caregivers, children look to us for guidance and it's up to us to lead the way.

Having said that, starting the conversation can be tough. If you're like most parents, you've done your homework and you'll know that there is a wealth of information available in books and on the Internet. So much so, that it's overwhelming and who has the time to sift through it all?

In addition, while there's an abundance of information, very little of it will teach you HOW to successfully communicate the information to your kids. Let's face it, children don't come with instruction manuals and as a parent, sometimes it's hard to know what to do. *What's appropriate? What's normal? What's not? What do I say? What do I do?*

To complicate matters, as adults we bring preconceptions and emotions surrounding our own experience with sexuality into the equation. Most of us have the best of intentions, but very few of us grew up in homes where talking about sex was as natural as talking about the weather.

We've consulted with experts, reviewed the literature extensively and distilled it into easy to read, manageable pieces along with talking points on how to **Start the Conversation** with your child.

Our goal is to help you, make those tough conversations easy so that you in turn can help your children to stay healthy and safe.

# TABLE OF CONTENTS

# STARTING THE CONVERSATION

*Sex Education: It's More Than Learning About How Babies Are Made!* Outlines behaviours that are typical for preschool children along with the information they should know as they grow through the ages of 2 to 5. It includes strategies for answering questions they might ask in an age appropriate way, tips on initiating conversations with young children about sexual health, along with resources to help take the stress out of doing both.

What can you expect from children ages 2-5?

## Curiosity

- *learning that bodies come in all shapes, sizes and colours*
- *noticing physical differences between boys and girls*
- *pregnancy and how babies are born*
- *touching their genitals*

What should you be encouraging in children ages 2-5?

## Realization

- *boys experience practice erections*
- *body parts have proper names*
- *boundaries exist and should be respected*
- *bodies are private and should be respected*
- *genders exist and they identify with one*
- *traditional gender roles exist and they recognize them*

# An Important Note!

Every child develops at their own rate, some earlier or later than others. No two children are exactly alike, each has their own personality and an approach that works for one, may not necessarily work for another. As their parent, you're in the best position to know what will. While these modules are designed as a support tool for the important discussions you'll have with your child, they are NOT rulebooks. Children don't always fit exactly into these age categories and the responsibility lies with you to gauge your child's emotional, mental and physical development in order to provide them with the correct information at the appropriate time.

# MAKING TOUGH CONVERSATIONS EASY

Not only does talking to young children about sexual health protect them from abuse, it also opens up the lines of communication between you and your child. Children are being exposed to sexual messages earlier and earlier and starting the conversation when they're young sets you up as their go to source for information on sexual health, not friends, the Internet or other less reliable sources. If you're concerned that talking about sex to your kids will have a detrimental effect, quite the opposite is true. Studies show that children who have been taught about sexuality from adults they trust wait longer to engage in sex, have fewer partners, and experience less incidences of teenage pregnancy and STI's. Another great benefit? If you can talk to your kids about sex, you can talk to them about anything!

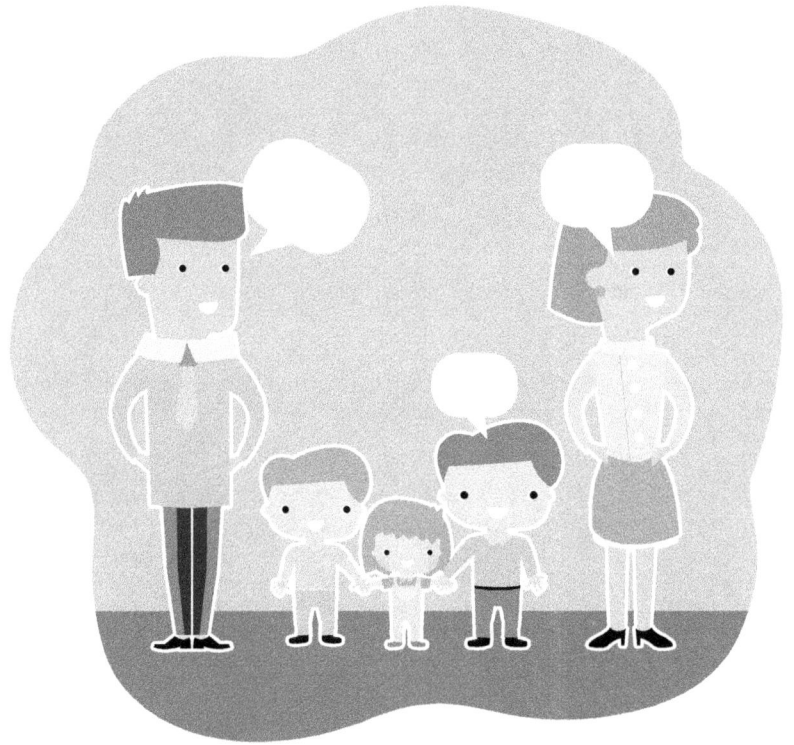

The good news is that this age group is the easiest to talk to because they haven't learned that sexuality is still a taboo subject in our society. This makes them very receptive to information.

## Strategies

If your child hasn't asked you questions about sexual health, don't wait for the perfect moment to have a discussion! As parents, it's up to you to start the conversation.

Children begin to show interest in their sexuality long before they're able to actually ask their questions and because your child's experience outside the home is limited at this age, their immediate family is their biggest influence. If you're stuck, don't be afraid to use ready-made scripts that explain concepts and answer questions in children's books movies and Apps. One of the best ways to initiate conversations is by addressing these topics while playing catch, doing dishes, riding bikes, or even driving in the car.

Ask your child open-ended questions and use supportive comments like:

- *How do you think it happens?*
- *What do you think?*
- *What a great question!*

Once you've initiated the conversation, be sure to keep it up! Since children in this age group only remember what they want to, you need to repeat the same conversations over and over... And over.

## How do I answer my child's questions?

First, clarify. Children in this age group are VERY literal. When your child asks you a question, clarify by responding with one of your own, such as:

- *What do you think?*
- *Where did you hear that?*
- *Why are you asking?*
- *Tell me more…*

Doing this allows you to find out where the question is coming from and what your child wants to know while also buying you time to phrase a thoughtful, appropriate response. Don't make this a more challenging job than it needs to be! Talking to your child about sexual health doesn't have to be difficult, all you need to do is stick to the facts, keep it simple and use the right scientific terminology.

## What topics are appropriate?

Basically, anything and everything they want to hear. Don't defer conversations about sexual health because you're afraid that they're too young to know. If they're asking questions, they're ready for answers. Keep in mind that these talks don't get easier as your child gets older. They get harder.

## How much information is enough?

Your child will let you know, as they'll change the subject or walk away when they've had enough.

## Lead by example!

The things you do and the way you act will influence your child's perception of love, affection, conflict resolution, and body image. From an early age, your child is learning from you, even when you're not actively teaching.

Your nonverbal cues (i.e. gestures, eye contact, body language) speak volumes about your comfort level and about your perceptions of sex and sexuality. Model the behavior you want your child to exhibit and commit to an honest, open dialogue about sexual health.

It's okay to feel embarrassed if you're initially uncomfortable having these conversations with your child. Most of us weren't raised in homes that encouraged open sexual dialogue. If your parents were uncomfortable talking to you about sex it's understandable that you in turn will be too. Don't let that put you off! A great way to begin is by practicing scientific names for body parts with your child and once you're comfortable, using them in conversation. You'll be amazed by how quickly it gets easier. Be kind to yourself if you stumble, the important thing is to keep trying! By the time you're raising a teenager, the same words that made you blush, will be rolling easily off your tongue.

Be patient! Answering questions repeatedly can be frustrating but isn't that part of being a parent? Treat every question they ask as a potential teaching moment. Take these opportunities when they present themselves and don't be discouraged if you have to repeat the same thing again and again. Children learn through repetition and evidence shows that many small conversations over time are way more beneficial than one long talk every now and then. Remember this information can't hurt them but it CAN protect them.

## BOTTOM LINE

- Communication is the key to becoming an approachable parent! It's okay to be uncomfortable, but starting the conversation is the most important thing. Rest assured, it will get easier over time.
- As parents, it's up to you to start the conversation. Starting the conversation early sets you up as their go to source for information on sexual health.
- When your child asks you a question, clarify by responding with one of your own.
- When explaining sexual health to your child, stick to the facts, keep it simple and use the right scientific terminology.
- Model the behaviour you want your child to exhibit and commit to an honest, open dialogue about sexual health.

*In the next section...*

*Small things can make a big difference! Once you've started the conversation, it's important to teach your child what their body parts are and how they work because it can protect them from abuse.*

# BODY TALK: PARTS & FUNCTIONS

As your child develops, they start to experience involuntary physical and emotional changes as their body responds to their external environment and their biology. Younger children in this age group begin noticing physical differences between girls and boys while children at the older end of the spectrum begin understanding that these differences are permanent. A little girl might wonder why she doesn't have a penis. A little boy might wonder why his penis looks different from his dad's.

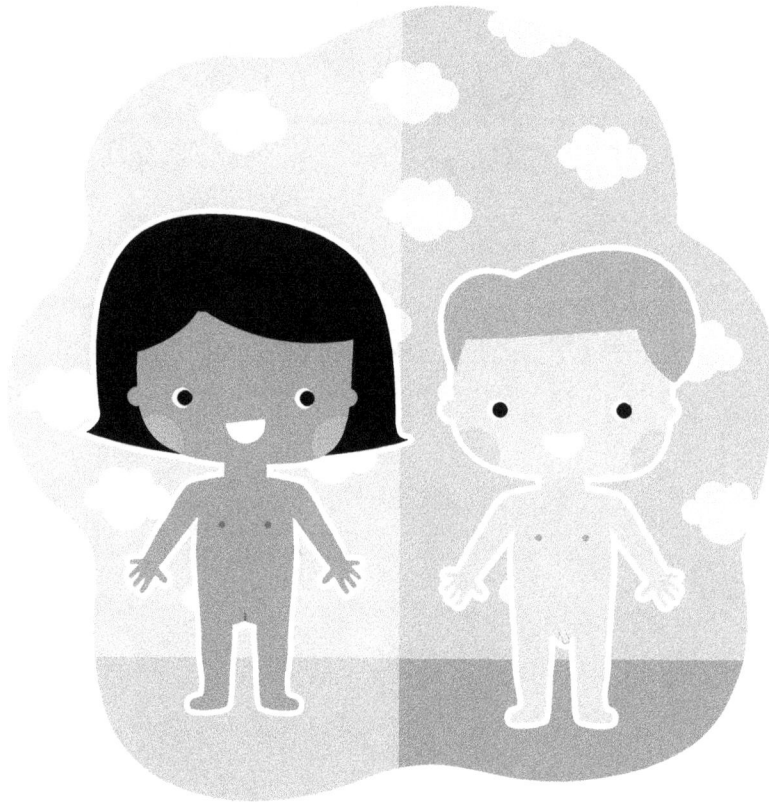

## What They Are

### How do I explain body parts?

Even if the words *penis, scrotum, vagina* or *labia* make you blush, try not to use nicknames or jargon! We've all used words like *pee pee* or *vajayjay*, but it's best to stick to the scientific names for body parts. Children who know what their body parts are and how they work are more protected from sexual abuse because predators recognize that these children have an open dialogue with their parents or caregivers and are more likely to report inappropriate behaviour to a trusted adult using proper terminology.

**The first thing most children notice is that girls have a vulva and boys have a penis.**
**Teach your children that girls have the following:**

- *vulva (labia)*
- *clitoris*
- *vagina*
- *anus*
- *urethra*
- *uterus*
- *ovaries*

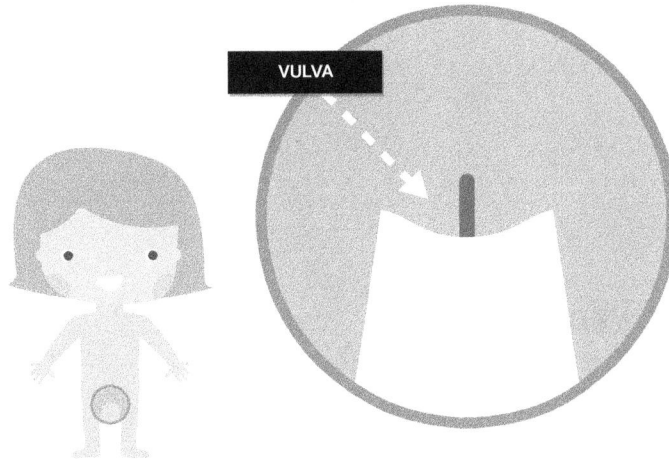

**Teach them that boys have the following:**

- *penis*
- *testicles*
- *scrotum*
- *urethra*
- *anus*

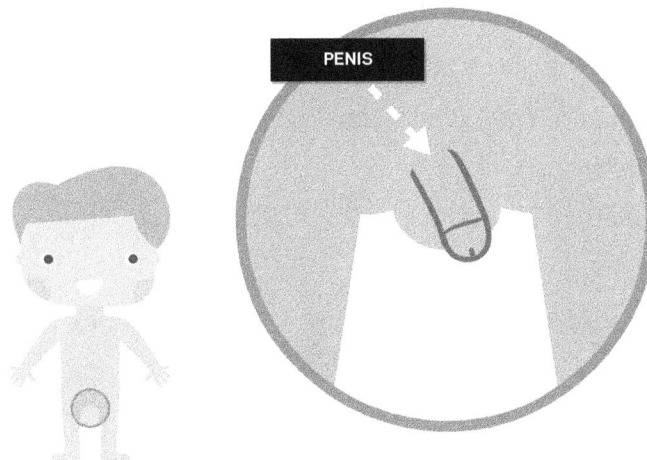

Bath time provides a great opportunity to identify their private parts in particular. Engage your child with open-ended questions, using the correct scientific terms. Remember: practice makes perfect! In addition, using the right words for private parts shows your child not only that you're not ashamed of your body, but that you're open to future conversations. Reinforce which body parts are private (*mouth, breasts and genitals*) so your child feels confident, comfortable, and safe disclosing inappropriate touching to you or another trusted adult.

START THE CONVERSATION...
• Do you know which body parts are private?
• How are a boy/girls parts different?
• Can you say the word?
• What makes them private?
• What makes private parts so special?

# How They Work

### How do I explain body functions?

Explain to your daughter that the skin between her legs is called the *vulva (or labia)*. At the front of the vulva is the *clitoris*, which looks like a tiny knob about as big as the end of a little finger. Show your daughter a picture to help her understand what her body looks like.

Explain to your daughter that girls have three openings between their legs:
- *vagina (where the baby enters the world from the uterus/womb)*
- *anus (where stool exits the body)*
- *urethra (where urine exits the body*

Teach your son that the body part hanging between his legs is called a *penis* (not wiener/dinky/dick) and that its purpose is to deliver sperm. Because the penis can only deliver sperm when it's erect, penises practice erections before boys are born and several times a day as they are growing up. You may hear comments like *Mommy, my penis is magic! It goes up and down!* Reassure your son that this is normal and a sign that his body is preparing for having a baby someday. (We deal with having babies in more detail in the chapter *Telling the Truth About How Babies are Made*).

Identify their *testicles* (not balls/nuts), explaining that they're carried in a bag of stretchy skin called the *scrotum* and their purpose is to make *sperm* as well as a substance called *testosterone* that helps boys grow into healthy adult men.

Explain that boys have two openings between their legs:

- *urethra at the tip of the penis (where urine exits the body)*
- *anus (where stool exits the body).*

Don't forget to teach your son about the female body and your daughter about the male body as well. Knowledge is empowerment and protection!

**START THE CONVERSATION ...**
- Do you know why boys have their testicles on the outside and girls have their ovaries on the inside?
- Can boys have babies? What do you think? Why? Why not?
- Can you tell me why girls have a womb and boys don't?
- What do you think?
- Why do you say that?

**Remember!**

While it's important to have a sense of humor when talking about body science, try not to laugh or giggle when discussing erections or other bodily functions. This communicates that you're not comfortable with the subject and will prompt your child to model your behaviour. It's okay to be embarrassed! Just try to keep the giggling to a minimum.

How you respond to your child's natural inquisitiveness will greatly influence their perceptions about body image and sexuality and also set the tone for their communication with you moving forward. Without this dialogue, questions may be answered by unsafe or unreliable sources.

# Keeping It Clean

It's never too early to talk to your children about genital hygiene!

Show your child how to clean their genitals just like you would if you were teaching them to

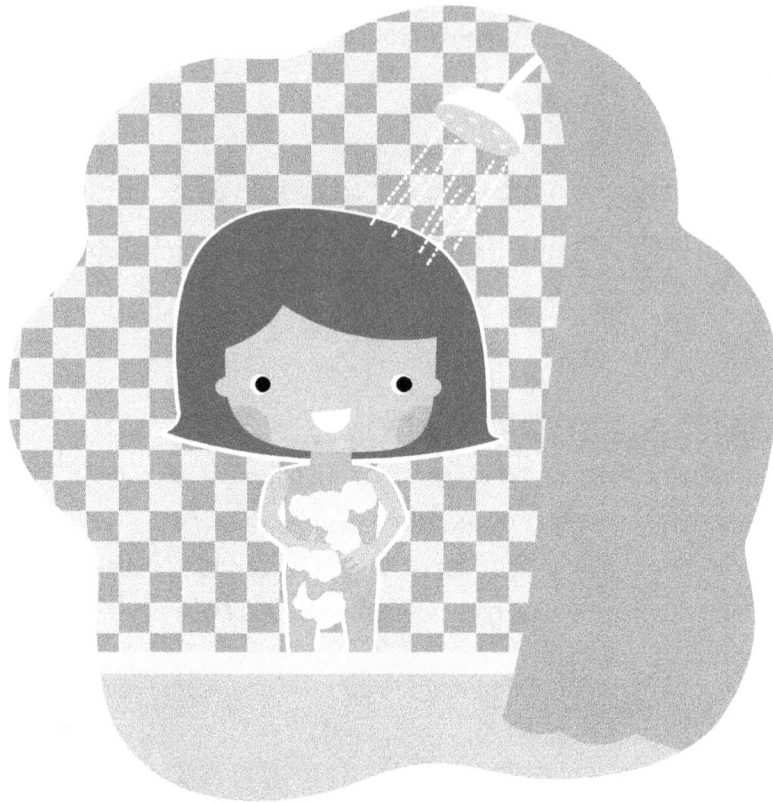

wash any other body part. When children are comfortable with their genitals, they'll be able to recognize and to tell you when something isn't right or if they have an infection. Teach your child to wash the smegma (a white, odorous substance) from under the skin of their penis or from between the folds of their vulva.

Don't assume that children intuitively know how to clean themselves. This is a skill that takes both direction and practice.

## START THE CONVERSATION ...
- Why do you think it's important to clean your private parts?
- Do you think it's a good idea for children to clean their private parts every day?

Teach your daughter to wipe down and away from the vulva, especially after a bowel movement, since stool can cause an infection if it enters the urethra. Teach your son that because testicles should be kept cool, it's wise for boys to sleep naked or in loose underwear.

**Although rare, intense testicular or abdominal pain can be the result of testicular torsion, which occurs when the testicles twist inside the scrotal sac. If this occurs, seek immediate medical attention.**

# Why Is My Penis Different?

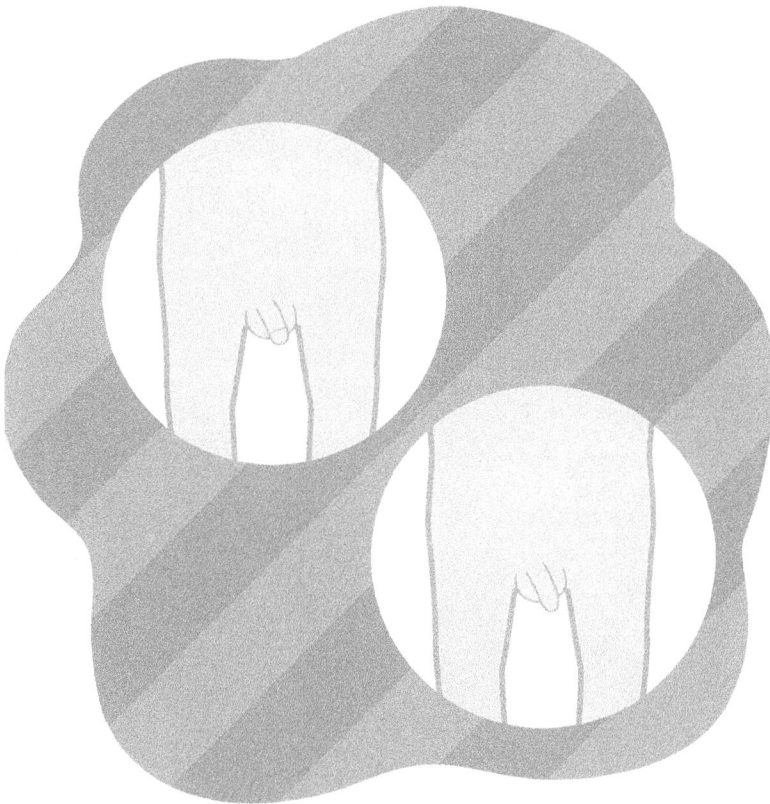

Your son may notice that his penis looks different or similar to other penises. He may also compare his penis specifically to his dad's penis and wonder why they look different.

Reassure him that although penises might look different, they all work the same way. Explain that when a baby is born, some families make the decision to remove the stretchy skin (the *foreskin*) that surrounds the tip of the penis but either way this doesn't affect the health, cleanliness or functionality of the penis. Don't avoid the circumcision discussion as it may lead to anxiety or feelings of alienation. You're the best person to explain why he was or wasn't circumcised.

**START THE CONVERSATION ...**
· What do you think of your penis?
· Have you seen/noticed penises that look different to yours?
· How are they different to yours?

# Going Potty

This is a great time to explain to your kids how their parts work and why each part has a different function.

Potty training typically occurs between 1.5 and 4 years of age. Children who are younger than eighteen months don't possess the muscle strength to control their bowel movements and urine flow. Although the duration of potty training varies, it typically takes several months from the time you properly introduce the process to your child. Children from ages 2-3 tend to be the easiest to train.

**Signs that your child may be ready for potty training:**

- *communicating prior to or after soiling their diaper*
- *using the terms pee/urine or poo/stool*
- *showing interest in the toilet/potty*
- *showing interest when you go to the toilet*
- *understanding simple questions like "Do you have to pee?"*
- *acting uncomfortable when their diaper is soiled*
- *exhibiting a desire for independence*
- *pulling their pants up and down*
- *not defecating during the night*
- *experiencing dry periods of at least 1-2 hours*
- *waking up dry from a nap*

**Teach me the basics!**

If you feel that your child is ready for potty training, there are several ways that you can make the transition easier.

- Allow your child to see you use the toilet so they become familiar with the routine of wiping, flushing, and hand washing.
- If you choose to train your child on a conventional toilet with a potty insert, be sure to provide a footstool so their feet are supported.
- Portable potties also have their benefits as they're convenient, accessible, and can be placed somewhere that keeps them front of mind.
- Teach your son to sit while he's learning to go potty. Only when he's gotten the hang of it

should you teach him how urinate standing up. Get him to aim at a Cheerio in the toilet bowl to teach aim and control.

- Source books and DVDs on the subject. Reading to children about potty training is a good way of enticing them to stay on the potty while also reinforcing the process.

## Pull-ups versus underwear: the pros and cons:

Pull-ups are easier to use and less messy, but they feel just like diapers. Underwear on the other hand, can be messier for the parent but the child will likely be more inclined to learn faster due to the discomfort (although this is not always the case). If you decide on underwear, let your child choose it for themselves. Bear in mind that summer is a good time for potty training since they'll have more opportunity to be naked.

## Be consistent!

Make the potty a part of the daily routine. Have your child sit on it at the same time everyday or regularly throughout the day, every two hours or so.

Track how often they *go* in their diaper to gauge when you should be putting them on the potty. Some children will warn you prior to *going* but it's more common for them to tell you after they've already *gone*. Regardless, always be positive and encouraging, positive reinforcement is important, whether it takes the form of sticker charts, treats, or just praise and smiles. Take your child's personality into account! They may become uncomfortable with too much praise, which could accomplish the opposite of what you're trying to achieve.

Negative behaviour will only backfire. This can be a frustrating process for them as well and reacting negatively to their failures can undermine their confidence. Remember to keep your emotions in check and respect your child's privacy.

It's not uncommon for children to remain in a diaper at night long after they've been potty trained in the day. Nighttime potty training tends to take longer since children sleep deeply and don't yet have the bladder control to last the whole night without going. You'll know they're ready for underwear at night when their diaper is dry in the morning. It may also be wise to minimize water consumption before bedtime. Be prepared, because most preschoolers are still getting the hang of using the toilet, it's common for the occasional nighttime accident to occur. When they do, relax! It's all a part of the process.

If your child doesn't want anything to do with potty training yet, put the potty away and try again after a few weeks. Don't pressure your child if they're not ready, being able to go to the bathroom at a young age is not reflective of intelligence.

**Try to avoid potty training during big transitions such as moving house or the arrival of a new sibling. It's common for children to completely regress with potty training when a new baby arrives. Have patience and try again after some time has passed.**

**Bed wetting again?**

**If your child suddenly begins having accidents long after staying dry all night, several factors could be responsible: Rule out urinary tract infection first by ensuring that the urine is clear, not cloudy or pink. If you suspect an infection, see your healthcare provider immediately. Sometimes, bed wetting can be due to emotional stimuli such as separation anxiety, changes in the family dynamic or abuse.**

Be careful not to force your child to kiss or hug someone whom they don't want to because it sends mixed messages and teaches them to ignore their instincts. A forced hug or kiss is disrespectful to the child. Instead, why not ask *Does Aunt Nancy get a hug today?* This empowers the child to make the decision. If it's a no hugs day, high fives and waves can take their place. Forcing a child to kiss someone against their will is asking them to use their mouth (a private part) against their will.

**START THE CONVERSATION ...**
- Do you know/remember what makes private parts so special?
- What does a good touch feel like? A hug from mom and dad?
- When is it okay for someone to touch another person? (E.g. Doctor's appointment or a mom changing a baby's diaper).
- Tell me about when you don't want to say hi to someone with a kiss and hug?
- How does that make you feel? Can you say why?
- What could you do instead of a hug or kiss?
- What can you say if you don't want to hug or kiss someone?
- It's important you listen to what your body says, hi fives or handshakes are good too.
- What do you think if an adult wants to touch a child?
- What do you think you should do if someone touches you in your private parts?

# Safety! 25 Things You Should Know!

**Knowledge is protection!**

The body boss and body boundaries lessons are important because they boost awareness, build confidence and most importantly, offer protection. As parents, our worst fear is having our child targeted by predators. Let's face it, the topic of sexual abuse is a sensitive one but when the stats are so staggering (1 out of 4 girls and 1 out of 6 boys will be sexually abused by age 18) it's not a topic that can be ignored. Keep in mind that 90 percent of those who abuse children are in and around the family, not strangers lurking in the sidelines. Take the following information to heart.

Regardless of who's committing the abuse, there are commonalities among all perpetrators:

Many perpetrators utilize what experts call the *grooming* process. Grooming (which usually starts well in advance of the act of abuse) is a gradual process that involves gaining the trust of both the child and their family. This is done to lower the child's inhibitions in preparation for sexual abuse. Children who know and trust an offender are much less likely to report the abuse. Predators prefer getting close to their victim's family because their proximity makes the child's story seem less believable if the abuse happens to be reported.

The labels vary, but most sexual abuse will involve the following 6 steps:

1. **Targeting the child**
2. **Gaining their trust**
3. **Filling a special need**
4. **Isolating the child from their peers**
5. **Sexualising the relationship, and finally**
6. **Maintaining control over the child.**

Most sexual offenders are quite calculating with their attention and affection and know exactly how to balance the way that they interact with the child in private and in public to avoid detection. Children who are being *groomed* by a predator will often idealize the offender, who *seduces* them into believing that they share a *special* relationship. This often leads to victims becoming willing participants in their own abuse.

When the trust of the child is gained, the abuser will start to desensitize the child to sexualising the relationship and make them believe that this is *normal* behaviour. Sexual offenders desensitize a child to the sexualising process by crossing the line bit by bit over time (e.g. walking in when they're dressing).

Once an offender has sexualized a relationship with a child, it's easier to manipulate the child's physical response, which reinforces the child's emotional attachment. Sexually abused children don't realize that their physical response to stimulation is beyond their control, which leads to feelings of guilt which the abuser in turn uses as leverage to manipulate the child into thinking that the abuse is their fault.

Sexual offenders keep children in an abusive relationship by using their own lack of self-esteem, guilt and emotional vulnerability against them. Abused children are often more afraid of the consequences of telling (isolation, humiliation) than suffering the ongoing abuse.

ALWAYS believe the child!

## 7 Things to look out for:

- Adults that seem to give more attention to children than other adults.
- Child molesters will seek out places children frequent (parks, sports grounds, shopping malls etc)
- Adults who like to be in physical contact with children a lot. i.e., tickling, wrestling and have children sit on their lap.
- An adult your child idealizes for reasons you DO NOT understand.
- An adult who is always finding reasons to be around and is always offering to watch the children.
- An adult in or around the family showing a child undue attention, giving them gifts or money for no apparent reason.
- Adults that try to make opportunities (babysitting, coaching, trips, sleepovers) to spend time alone with your child.

## 11 Signs of abuse:

- Is the child afraid of a family member or another adult? Investigate!
- Is the child behaving in a sexual manner that is not age appropriate?
- Is the child exhibiting behaviour that is not developmentally appropriate? Ask questions and investigate.
- Is there blood in the child's underwear or do they have chronic bladder infections?
- Does the child act secretive about the unexplained acquisition of gifts/toys?

- Do they masturbate excessively? It may be innocent but it's worth looking at closer.
- The child tells you that they have a *secret* and *can't tell*.
- Exhibiting regressive behaviour such as thumb sucking.
- The child acting out sexually with toys or inserting foreign objects into their vagina or anus.
- Night terrors and soiling the bed after being potty trained. Many children can demonstrate this for various reasons, but its worth looking into if it becomes more common.
- Unexplained behaviour such as incessantly crying and clinginess for no reason. Ask questions and investigate.

Don't forget to emphasize that when secret touching happens, it's never the child's fault.

### START THE CONVERSATION ...
- Explain to your child that some adults have touching problems and they touch children's private parts when they're not supposed to. These people are sick and need help. Ask:
- Do you know anyone with a touching problem?
- What is an example of a good secret? A bad secret?
- What do you think about when touching is a secret?
- What do you think about adult and children touching or kissing each other's private parts?
- What should you do if someone asks you to touch someone else's private parts?

## Feeling Things Out

Its important to know that self-stimulation is a perfectly normal part of development throughout childhood and into adulthood. Masturbation is healthy, exploratory behaviour that children do in order to feel pleasure, experience comfort or sometimes just out of curiosity and boredom. Don't be surprised if your daughter or son is playing with their genitals.

## Take a deep breath!

Acknowledge that it's fine for them to touch themselves providing they're alone in the bedroom or bathroom (because children often touch themselves in public, it's important to remind them that their genitals are private).

Once your message has been conveyed, distraction is an effective exit strategy in this age group. Take these opportunities when they present themselves, lessons like this often bear repeating!

## What if I discover my child exploring with another child?

Children's tendency to *play doctor* is prompted by the need to physically compare themselves with other children of both sexes and is common between children of the same age group. If an older child is involved, the behaviour needs to be stopped immediately and closely monitored. If you encounter this scenario, calmly ask your child to get dressed, reminding them that their private parts are special and need to be kept private from other people. Later, initiate a more detailed conversation in which you identify the private parts (*mouth, breasts, genitals*) by their scientific names and answer any questions that arise from the discussion. Be sure to afford the older child the same respect and dignity you would the younger.

To preempt this behaviour, instate an open door policy at home and on play-dates.

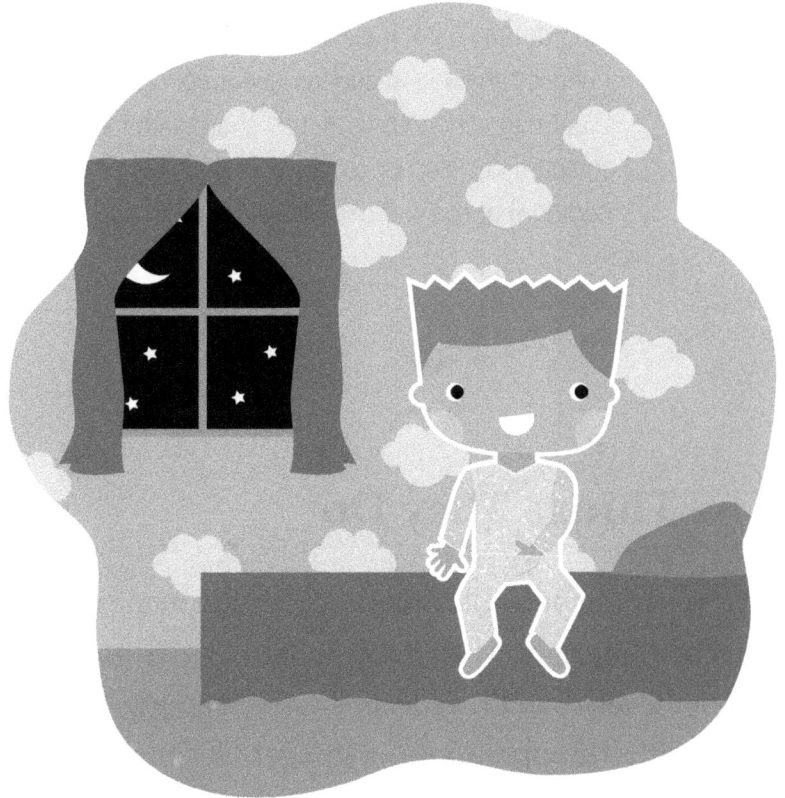

**START THE CONVERSATION ...**
- Do you know what private/public means?
- Where is it appropriate to touch yourself (Bedroom/bathroom)?
- Do you know what private is/means?
- I know it feels good when you touch yourself but do you know where is it appropriate to do so?
- Why do you think it's important to keep it private?
- I understand you're curious about how other people bodies look, like (insert child's name). What interests you? Can you share with me what you want to know? It's not appropriate to share our own or touch other people's private parts, because they are special to the person that owns them. Please come to me and I'll help you with what you want to know.

# The Things They Do

You've taught your child the appropriate names for their body parts which is a step in the right direction but right when you're about to give yourself a pat on the back, they start running down the aisles in the grocery store screaming *Vagina! Vulva! Penis!* Was it a mistake to arm them with the appropriate language? Of course not! It's just time to redirect that excitement to a more appropriate setting: the home.

Teaching your child about appropriate behaviour, good manners, privacy, and boundaries empowers them to show respect for themselves and others. Tell your child that you're happy they're able to express themselves using the appropriate scientific names for their body parts and remind them that their bodies are indeed something to be proud of. Explain that it's not appropriate to show or discuss private parts in public because private means that they are not for other people to see, touch or kiss.

**Don't avoid this conversation or leave it for when your child starts asking questions or enters school.**

Try not to yell at or shame your child. Obviously, you can't ignore inappropriate behaviour but using language like dirty, not normal or bad will just give them a negative perception of their body and their curiosity surrounding it. Berating or punishing only tells them that what they're feeling is shameful and wrong. Remember, how you respond to your child's natural inquisitiveness will greatly influence their perceptions of body and sexuality plus shape the tone of your future dialogue and without this dialogue, questions may be answered by unsafe or unreliable sources.

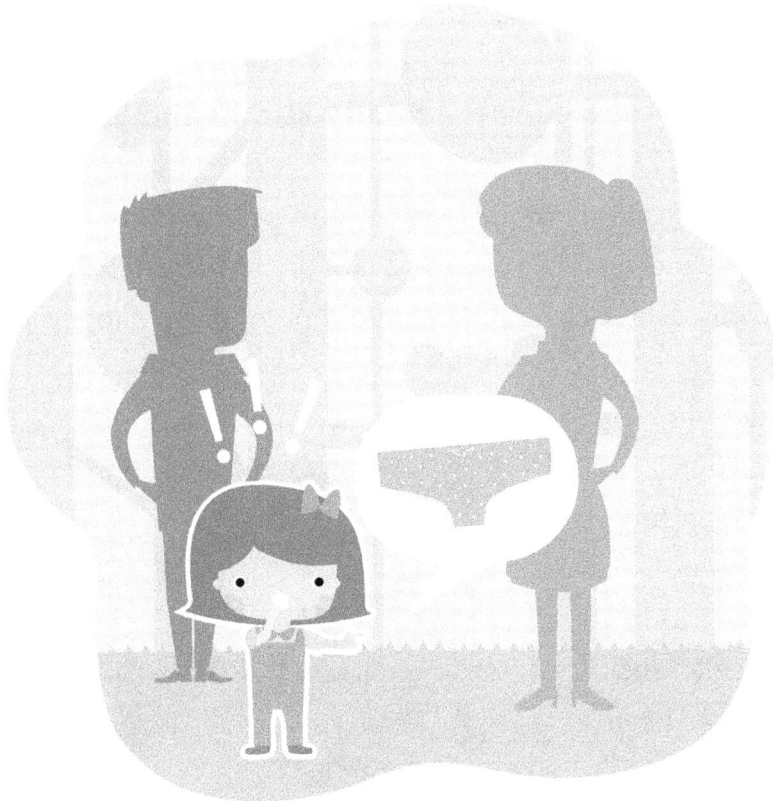

## START THE CONVERSATION ...
- What makes you happy about your body? Reinforce the positive.
- Why are private parts private? Reinforce that they are special to the person that owns them.
- Do you think it's proper to discuss private parts with others outside the home? Why?
- When we talk about private parts it's important we don't share that information with other people. Do you know why?

# The Rules of Engagement

Most parents are familiar with stranger danger. The idea that individuals are lurking in the shadows waiting to snatch your child the minute you turn around is every parents' worst nightmare. Society has become hypersensitive to this notion but statistically only a small percentage of children are harmed by strangers.

**90% of abuse is committed by someone the family knows and 50% of abusers are family members.**

Nevertheless, vigilance and education are the best ways to protect your child and make them aware of their own safety. It's impossible to anticipate every situation that your child may encounter but there are still ways you can help them avoid potentially dangerous situations.

Teach your child to stay close in busy environments such as playgrounds, fairs, parks, and shopping malls and let them know it's imperative that they're always within visual range. Provide strategies and procedures to implement if they get lost. If they're in a mall or a built-up area, tell them to approach a shopkeeper and report that they're lost. If they're outdoors or away from developed areas, tell them to stay put. When you realize your child is lost, report it immediately to security personnel or a staff member as most buildings have a protocol for these situations.

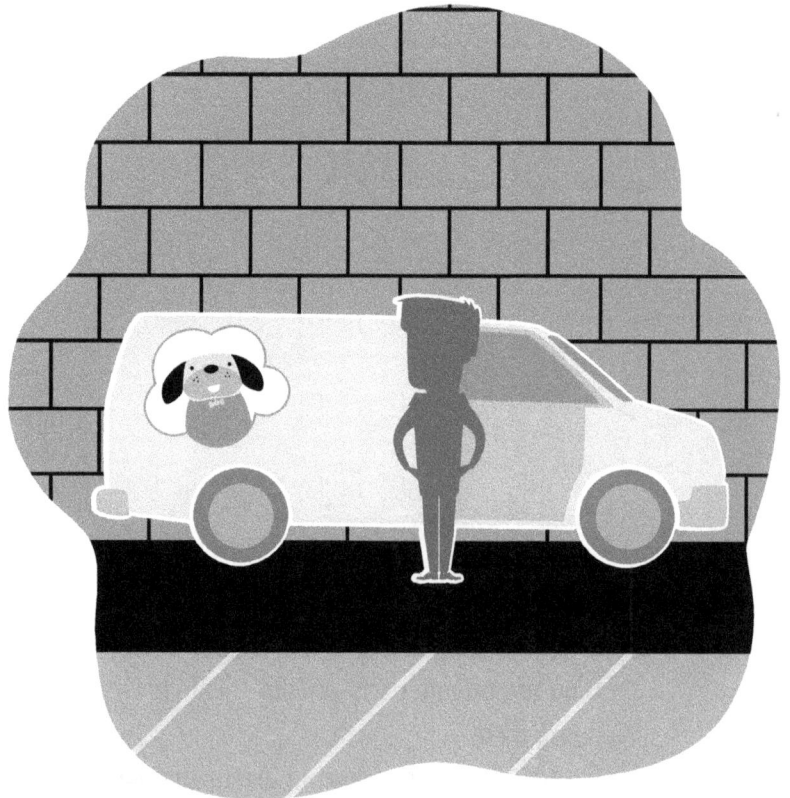

Have your child memorize their address and phone number and teach them how to use 911 (your regional emergency number) in the event of an emergency. Repetitively reinforce that it's never appropriate to speak to strangers beyond acceptable polite conversation.

Remind them to seek the help of a trusted adult if they're lost or need help and teach them to trust their instincts.

Provide them with examples of how a stranger might attempt to get their attention (e.g. candy, puppies, toys). Some ploys are more nefarious. Some strangers may ask for their help or say that they're friends with their parents. Teach your child to NEVER go anywhere with a stranger. Give them a codeword or phrase that only you or someone you trust would know, instructing them to NEVER go anywhere with someone who doesn't know it.

Conversely, it's important not to instill paranoia. It's critical that they understand each of these situations and know not to judge a book by its cover. Remind your child that strangers can also be kind, friendly and helpful. It's not about being afraid of strangers. It's about knowing the rules for interacting with them. Arming your child with the right tools will help them remain safe and empower them to say NO when strangers attempt to engage them.

## START THE CONVERSATION ...

- What is a stranger? What do they look like?
- Can you think of different types of trusted adults?
- If a stranger was knocking on the door, would you answer?
- If you are lost, who is a trusted adult you could go to in public? Police officer?
- If you are lost would you know what to do?
- Can you tell me other people who wear a uniform who aren't police officers?
- Can you think of a special (code) word that we could have together?
- What should you do/say if the stranger doesn't know the code word?
- Can you think of things the stranger might say if they don't know the code word to make you go with them?
- Do you think it's okay to say hello/goodbye to a stranger?
- When is it not okay to talk to a stranger?
- What do you say when that happens?
- Is it okay to accept gifts from strangers if it doesn't feel right?
- What would you say to the stranger?
- Do you think it's better for a child to help an adult, or for an adult to help an adult?
- What should you do if an adult asks you to help them and there is no adult around to help?

## BOTTOM LINE:

- Not only does your child need to understand the names and functions of their private parts. They need to learn their rights and identify their boundaries as well.
- Explain that it's inappropriate for anyone to touch or kiss their private parts or for them to touch or kiss the private parts of others.
- Make sure they understand that if anyone tells them this behaviour is okay or to keep it a secret, that it's wrong.
- Sexual abuse is a sensitive topic. It's more common than most people think so being educated on what to look for is important.
- Self-stimulation and exploration is completely normal and healthy behaviour that should be done in private, not public.
- Exploration with other children is normal for this age but children should be reminded that their private parts are special and shouldn't be shared.
- Only a small percentage of children are harmed by strangers but it's important to arm your children with the tools to protect themselves and stay safe.

*In the next section....*

*Once they understand that there are physical differences between sexes, children start to identify themselves as being male or female and realize that they're expected to behave in certain ways based on their gender. However, not all children fit neatly into stereotypical gender roles.*

# GIRLS VS BOYS

Children of this age start to notice the physical differences between males and females but their perceptions of gender roles are also being shaped by the far subtler messaging from society, culture, and media. When children begin to internalize these messages they start identifying themselves as male or female beyond their genitalia and attaching criteria for how girls and boys should behave.

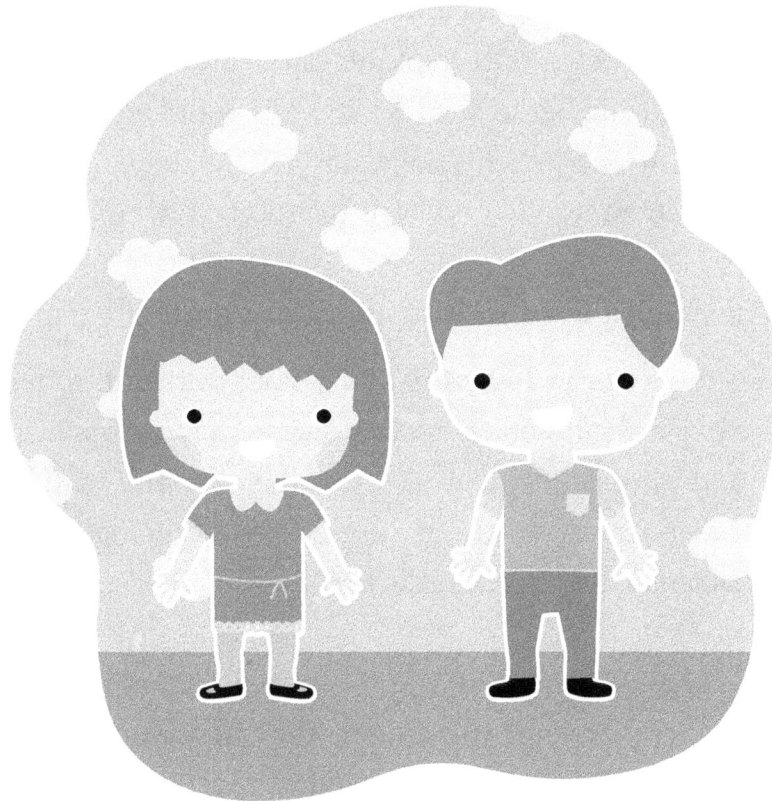

Parents of daughters know how difficult it is to avoid the barrage of princesses, pink, and all things pretty. Conversely, superheroes (accompanied by messages of toughness, strength and emotional suppression) dominate boys' toys. Even seasoned parents can be unaware of the gender stereotypes they can unintentionally reinforce in their children.

**Acknowledge your child's strengths and encourage, support, and celebrate them as an individual, not as a boy or a girl.**

From an early age, your child is learning from you, even when you're not actively teaching. As you model positive behaviours, you influence your child's perceptions and instill in them the morals and values you hold. Ultimately, children will follow what you're doing, not what you're saying. Lead by example!

## What strategies can I use to address stereotypes?

Encourage your child to treat others as individuals, correcting them if they make gender-specific statements. Encourage mixed play dates and activities that your child enjoys, regardless of their gender. Don't try to make your child conform to a particular stereotype. If your daughter isn't comfortable wearing dresses but opts for pants and a tee shirt instead, support her unique personality rather than pressuring her to *dress like a girl*. If your son likes dressing in girl's shoes and loves it when his sister paints his nails, don't make disparaging remarks. Children enjoy experimenting with different roles and need the room and support to do so.

## What if my child is having trouble embracing their gender?

Sometimes, children as young as age 2 identify as a gender different from their genitalia. It's common for children to experiment with different roles as they rationalize the world and their place in it but if your child consistently expresses that they identify with the gender opposite to their genitalia, they may be *transgendered* or a *gender-variant*. Being transgendered has nothing to do with *sexual orientation*. It simply means that the child feels different from the biologic sex they're supposed to be.

People who are gender-variants do not conform to any gender and have behaviours and interests that don't typically align with a specific gender. They may enjoy being a girl one day and a boy the next. Some children don't have a connection to either gender, which can be even more confusing.

## It's not a choice to be transgendered or a gender-variant person!

People are born that way. Being a transgendered or a gender-variant boy can be particularly hard since societal norms tend to be less flexible for males. A girl with a short haircut and boys clothes blends in much better than a boy with long hair and a dress.

The following 4 behaviours (when all present) can indicate that a child may be transgendered or a gender-variant:

- *bathroom behaviour (female child standing up to urinate)*
- *swimsuit aversion (trans children avoid swimsuits of their biological sex)*
- *type and style of desired underpants*
- *a strong desire to play with toys that are typically used by the opposite sex*

Suspecting that your child is transgendered or a gender variant can be very upsetting for a parent. You may experience the urge to change their behaviour but this can lead to shame, violence and embarrassment as the child gets older. Forcing them to be something they're not or ignoring who they are will have detrimental effects on their self-esteem, sense of self-worth, and overall happiness. They may see themselves as *unnatural* and experience overwhelming feelings of isolation.

It's important that the whole family seek support through this transition. The road to acceptance and unconditional love can be a long, painful one for all involved but for the sake of the child it must not be ignored.

**If you're having a hard time dealing with this, seek support and someone to talk to.**

## START THE CONVERSATION ...
- Do you think boys can wear pink? Can girls can play with trucks?
- What's your favourite colour?
- What's your favourite toy?
- How do you think boys and girls are different?
- What do you think is special about being a boy or girl? Tell your child how they are special in their own way.

## BOTTOM LINE

- Don't force your child to conform to stereotypes.
- Celebrate your child as an individual and encourage them to do the same.
- Forcing a child to be something they're not or failing to acknowledge them for who they are can have a negative effect on their sense of self worth.
- Transgendered or gender variant children are born that way.
- Transgendered children do not identify with the sex they were born into.
- Gender variant children do not identify with either male or female gender.

*In the next section....*

*This can be a very confusing time for children, because not only are they dealing with physical and behavioural changes, they also start to see differences in relationships between families, friends, siblings and others and question how they fit in.*

# MAKING CONNECTIONS

Parents and siblings are the key influencers in children's lives as they learn their family's dynamic and discover their role in it. Whether experiencing curiosity about their bodies, negotiating new friendships or grappling with divorce, it's important that you're aware of their thoughts and feelings.

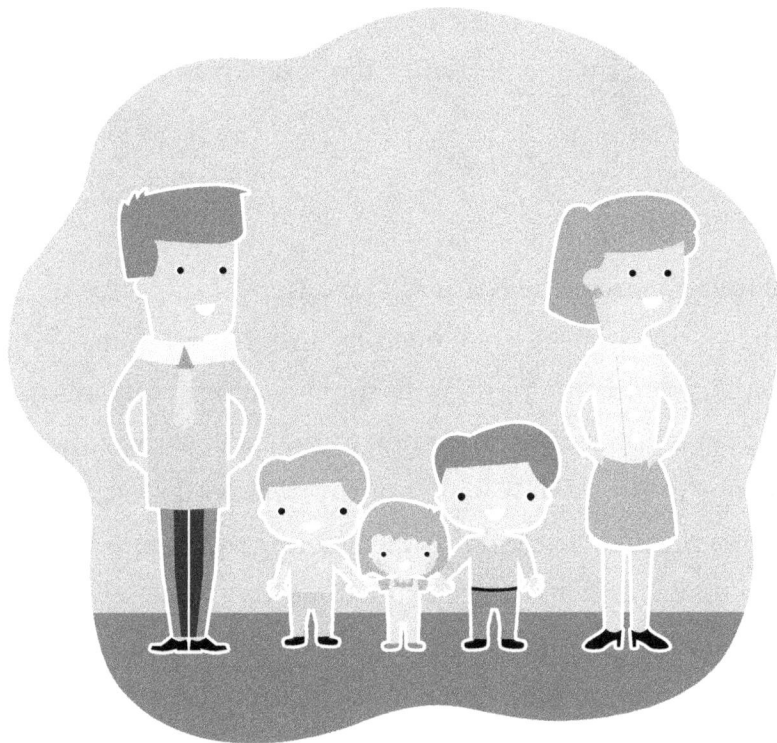

## Family Diversity

Just because children in this age group aren't capable of fully articulating their questions doesn't mean they aren't aware of their family's dynamic and inquisitive about that of other families. Explain to your child that every family is unique, made up of people who love one another regardless of the circumstances that created them. Celebrate these differences with your child! Families come in different shapes, sizes and forms. Some have a male and female parent while others have one parent, two same-sex parents, or even other family members acting as parents. Children are unique too. Some are biologically connected to their families while others are adopted or fostered. It's important to remember that all families are equal because they are composed of people who love and care for one another regardless of sexual orientation, age, race, gender, culture, or religion.

**Never express negative ideas about other family dynamics!**

**Every family has the same value providing its children are surrounded by love and stability. Most value judgments are based in fear or ignorance - two destructive qualities that no parent wants to nurture in their child!**

# Dealing With Divorce & Separation

Separation and divorce can be very traumatic for children because they learn far more from your actions and attitudes than you realize. Seeing parents in emotional conflict can be devastating for a child and have far reaching effects on how they view relationships throughout their lives. Parents who are going through a divorce are often so involved in their own misery that they can overlook the fact that their child may feel that they did or didn't do something to cause the split. Children aren't equipped to understand why their parents no longer want to be together and often fear that they will be abandoned by one parent or that one loves them less than the other.

**Divorce isn't about you. It's about your children.**

Reassure your child that both parents still love them and will always be a part of their lives (provided that's the case). Regardless of the circumstances, they need to understand that what's occurring isn't their fault. If possible, have this dialogue with them as a united front, no matter how painful it may be. Keep the conversation simple and stick to the facts, letting them know what to expect and answering questions in a way that's age appropriate while respectful to your privacy too. Allowing your child to express their thoughts and feelings will help them make sense of the situation and help you to dispel any misconceptions that may arise.

Children find it hard to adapt to a new family dynamic when one or both parents remarry, especially if the transition involves step-siblings. If you have a new partner, be patient if your child doesn't fall in love with them (and theirs) immediately. As far as they're concerned, this person is a stranger and you'll need to give your child time to get to know and trust them.

Be sensitive to the reality that children can often experience anger toward one or both parents for the divorce or separation and it may be hard for them to see you move on (particularly if they secretly harbor hopes of seeing their parents reunite).

Don't blame or malign your ex-partner in front of your child, even if you feel that you're the wronged party. All your child wants is to take your pain away. If you ignore the high road, they'll only take on your negativity, which will affect everyone's relationships moving forward. Remember that your child is your child, not your confidant. Don't rely on them for emotional support, counsel or as a shoulder to cry on.

# Sisters & Brothers

Children turn to those closest to them for guidance, and the relationships they forge with siblings can set the stage for their behaviour in other relationships. Older siblings can often impart wisdom about family values and sexual/social interactions while younger ones can teach empathy. Fighting between siblings is normal and altercation is an excellent opportunity for teaching moments about conflict resolution but it's important to monitor their behaviour and pre-empt power imbalances to avoid bullying or physical abuse. Unlike sibling squabbling, bullying involves power imbalance, repetition, and a negative emotional response on the part of the victim. Parents must remain vigilant in order to differentiate between the two and act accordingly.

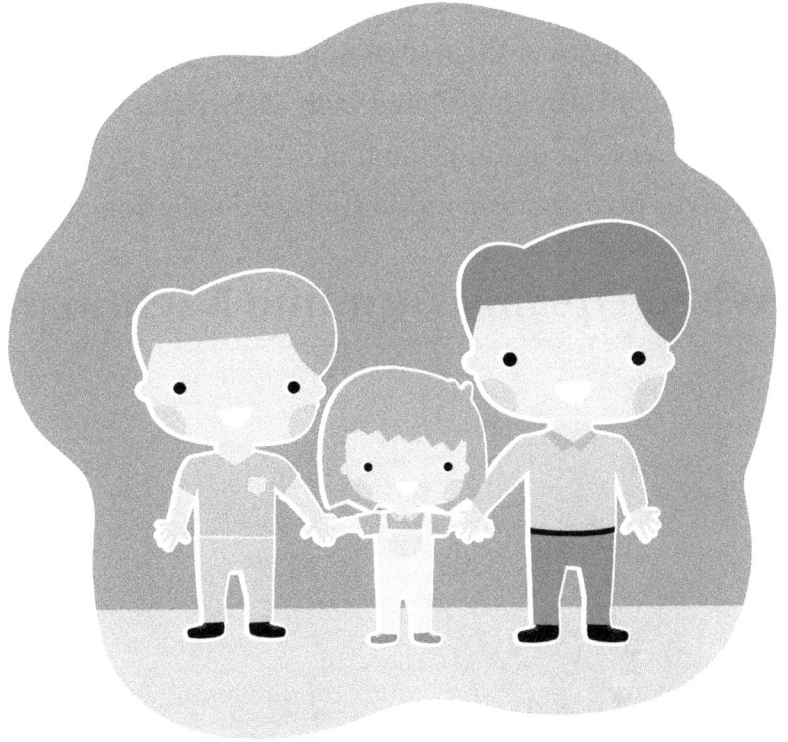

# My BFF

Often, children in this age group are in daycare or at preschool. This is when they begin playing in groups, forming opinions about whom they like playing with and developing friendships based on those feelings. Support your child as they forge new friendships through participation in social activities. Remember that the skill of relationship building is much easier for some children than others. Support their uniqueness and strive to make their environment comfortable, watching their interactions and stepping in when necessary to reinforce messages of sharing, caring, and empathy. Don't force your child into uncomfortable social situations. Anxious children take longer to warm up to other children and may benefit more from one-on-one play-dates in a quiet playground or backyard.

Family circumstances differ for every child, one parent may practice attachment parenting never leaving their child's side, while another may work full-time and employ a nanny. Your child's social development may vary depending on their exposure to other children and adults. Encourage supervised independence. By exercising due diligence with situations involving new individuals and scenarios, you give your child the opportunity to grow without continually hovering over them. Just make sure that the environment is controlled and that your child knows to inform you immediately if they feel unsafe.

Don't make the assumption that others share your values, sometimes, active, aware parenting involves investigating individuals and situations in which your child may come into contact.

# When Dreams Turn Into Nightmares

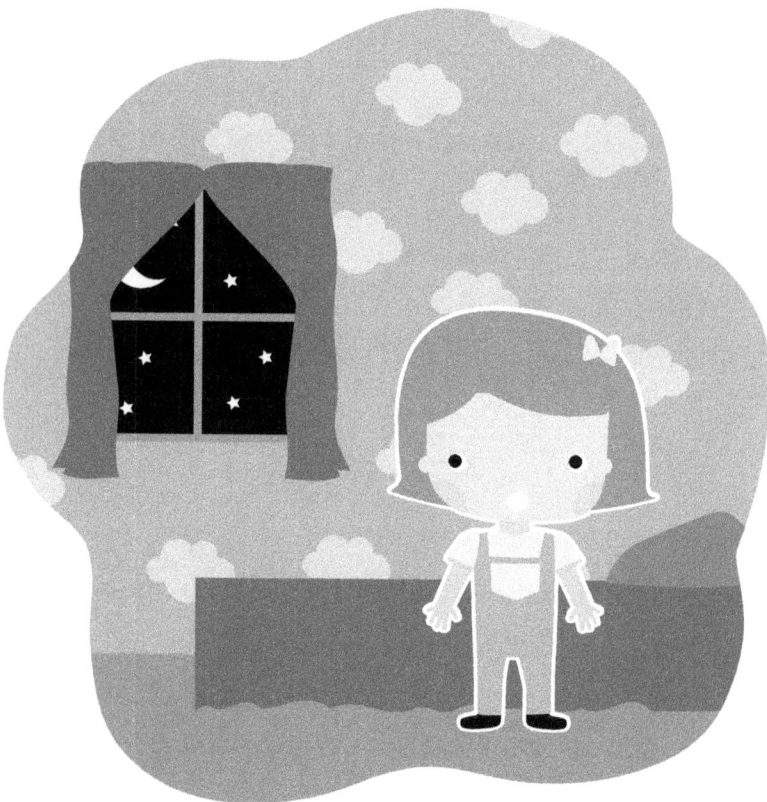

Dreaming is our brain's way of processing emotions and experiences but sometimes their subject matter turns them into nightmares. Nightmares can't always be attributed to a specific reason but in children, they can be catalyzed by factors as simple as change or stress.

When your child is awoken by a nightmare, reassure them that you're there and that what they experienced didn't happen in the real world. Offer comfort, showing them that you understand they're afraid and reassure them that feeling this emotion is fine. Remember to listen to your child because it helps them feel calm, safe, and protected. Install a night-light or hall light to allay anxiety as they fall back to sleep.

**If nightmares begin inhibiting your child from getting enough sleep or occur in concert with other behavioural problems, consult your doctor.**

Don't be dismissive or tell them to toughen up and go back to sleep. In a nightmare situation the child needs the comfort of knowing that they're safe and cared for.

## What about night terrors?

Night terrors are a little less common but often affect younger children. Usually occurring a few hours after the child falls asleep, they involve the child waking up and screaming for no apparent reason. Although seemingly awake, they in fact are not and typically don't respond to reassurance or touch.

When your child experiences a night terror, the best thing to do is simply ride it out. This can be upsetting for a parent but your job in this scenario is to make sure that they are in a safe environment. Children in this state can't be reasoned with but they will eventually settle down and go back to sleep.

**START THE CONVERSATION ...**
- What makes up a family?
- What do you love about your family?
- How do you feel about a family having only a dad or mom, grandparents etc? Talk about their feelings, explore.
- People come in all shapes, sizes and colors. Tell me about all the friends in your life and how they are different?
- How are they the same?
- Do you think their insides are the same as yours?
- How do you feel about mommy/daddy not being together any more? Why? Reinforce that you love them and that you understand what they're feeling.
- What do you think about mommy/daddy getting married to/living with someone else? Reinforce that they are special and will always be a part of your family.

## BOTTOM LINE:

- Every family is unique, made up of people who love one another regardless of the circumstances that created them.
- Divorce isn't about you. It's about your children.
- Unlike sibling squabbling, bullying involves power imbalance, repetition, and a negative emotional response on the part of the victim.
- Support your child as they forge new friendships through participation in social activities.
- Nightmares can't always be attributed to a specific reason but can be catalyzed by factors as simple as change or stress.

*In the next section....*

*What you've all been waiting for.... What to tell your Preschool children about the Birds and the Bees....*

# THE TRUTH ABOUT HOW BABIES ARE MADE

It's likely that by this age, your child has asked you the dreaded question *Where did I/do babies come from? Or How are babies made?*

Many parents are concerned that sexually educating their child at a young age leads to early sexual activity or promiscuity later in life. However, studies show that children who are taught about sex early tend to delay sexual activity. It's ignorance coupled with curiosity (not knowledge) that leads to earlier sexual experimentation. **Remember, children who have been taught about sexuality from reliable adults wait longer to engage in sex, have fewer partners, and experience less incidences of teenage pregnancy and STI's.**

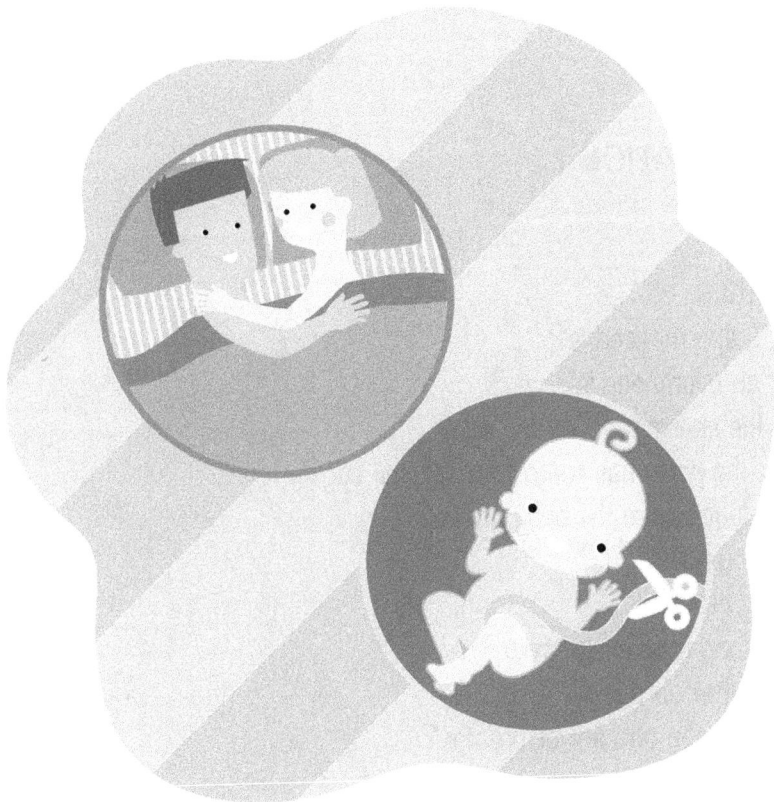

**Tell the truth!**

Babies don't come from the hospital or the stork! Explain the basics of reproduction, going into as much detail as you are comfortable with and watching for cues from your child that indicate their curiosity has been satisfied.

Start by explaining that a baby is made when a man's sperm (seed) is joined with a woman's ovum (egg) and starts to grow in her uterus or womb. Remember to use the scientific words for the body parts. If your child's reaction indicates that they're ready for more information, explain that in order for the sperm to mix with the ovum, the man usually puts his penis into the woman's vagina. As the baby grows in the womb it is surrounded by water (amniotic fluid) which protects the baby. The umbilical cord attaches from the mommy to the baby. This is how the mommy gives the baby the food it needs to grow and helps it "breathe".

When the baby is ready to be born, the mother's womb starts to push down around the baby (contract) like a great big hug to help it to move through the vagina (which stretches like an elastic to let the baby through and then goes back to it's normal size) and come out of the mother's body on a water slide. Sometimes, the doctor does an operation called a Cesarean or C-section to get the baby out instead. Once the baby is out of the mother's body, the doctor will cut the cord (which doesn't hurt the mom or the baby). After a few days the little bit of cord that was left falls off the baby and leaves a belly button behind.

This discussion is a basic introduction to answering questions on how babies are made. Our section on *Quick Answers for Kids* has the answers to additional questions your kids might have about reproduction and childbirth.

### START THE CONVERSATION ...
- Why do you ask?
- What do you think?
- What have you heard?
- What do you think a sperm/seed is?
- What do you think an ovum/egg is?
- How do you think the sperm reaches the egg?
- Where do you think the penis has to go to reach the egg?
- Can you name the place where the baby grows?
- What questions do you have?
- Where does the baby grow?
- Can you guess how long it takes to grow?
- Can you guess what that cord is for?
- How do you think the baby can eat or breathe?

# The Condom Conversation

Unfortunately, it's all too common to find used condoms in places like playgrounds and parks. It's important that children understand what they are and why they can't touch them. Use the prevalence of condom advertisements in the media as an opportunity for a teachable moment about this subject. Show your child how condoms look. Teach them that condoms allow adults to have sex without making a baby while also stopping the spread of germs from one person to another. Explain that they are clean and healthy when adults buy them from the store but have germs on them after they've been used. Because germs make people sick, children mustn't pick up condoms. If they find one, it's important that they know to report it to a trusted adult immediately.

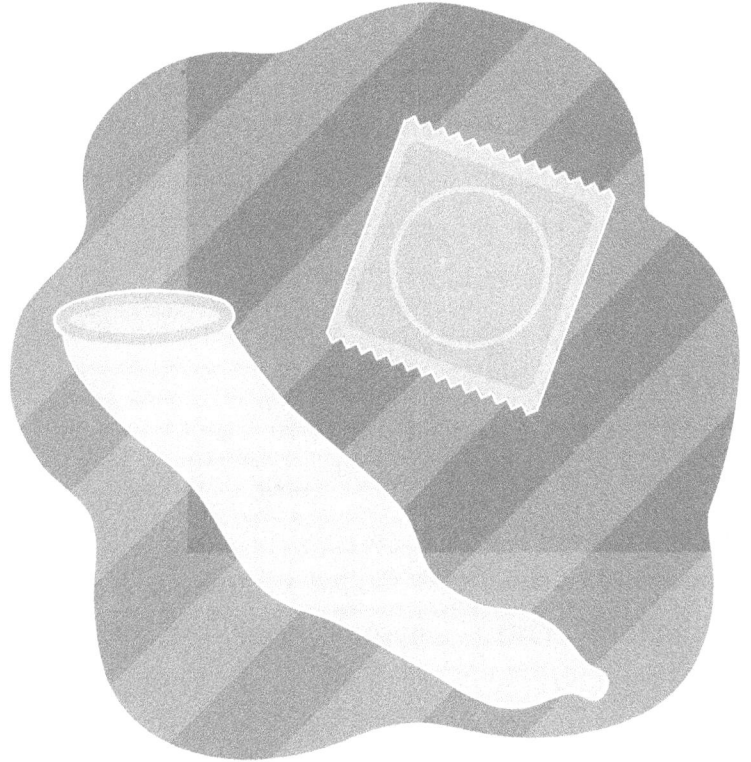

**Skipping the condom conversation can put your child at risk!**

Many viruses can live in dried bodily fluids for a long time. If your child thinks a condom is a balloon, they may handle it or even blow it up.

### START THE CONVERSATION ...
- Have you seen this in a park or playground before? Show picture of a condom
- What should you do if you see it?
- Why do you think it's important not to touch it? (Bad germs or bugs)
- What do you think it's used for?
- Is it clean in it's package?

# Relax! It's Only A Period

Children are inundated with feminine hygiene commercials on the television, come across products around the house and may even be in the bathroom when a parent's having her period. So, it's not surprising that they're curious about menstruation. If they ask what a period is, let your child know that when a girl is 12 or 13 (although it's normal for this to occur earlier or later) her body will begin practicing for pregnancy. Once a month when this happens, her uterus grows a lining and when she doesn't get pregnant, this lining leaves the uterus via the vagina in the form of drips. These drips look like blood but they're actually mostly water and tiny bits of skin. Most periods occur monthly and the drips last for about a week at a time.

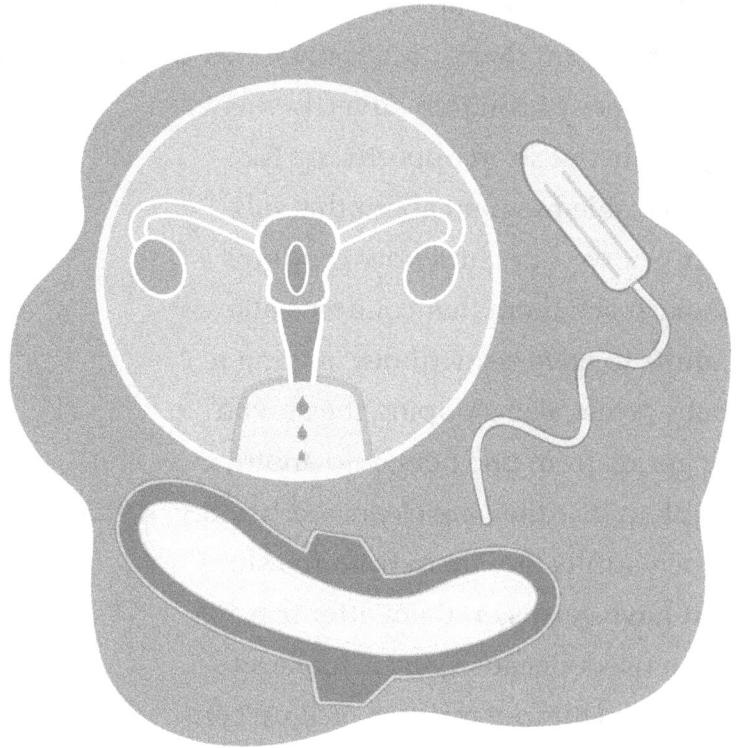

## START THE CONVERSATION ...
- Where do you think the blood comes from? It's not all blood, let me explain..
- Why do you think girls have their periods?
- Do you think it happens to both boys and girls?
- When do you think it happens? (Puberty)
- How do you feel about it?
- Does it scare you? Explain that it doesn't hurt
- Do you think it's normal? Explain that it's normal and all girls go through it.
- What do you think catches the drips when they come out of the body?
- How do you think a tampon (show picture) catches the drips?
- How do you think a pad (show picture) can be used to catch drips?

Don't skip this conversation or say *I'll tell you when you're older*. The visibility of feminine products makes this one of the easiest teachable moments to have!

## BOTTOM LINE:

- Studies show that children who are taught about sex early by a trusted adult tend to delay sexual activity later in life.
- When talking to your child about reproduction, be honest and stick to the facts. Eventually they're going to learn the truth and being less than honest undermines their trust in you.
- Children need to know what condoms look like and not to pick up them up, because they could contain harmful germs.
- Menstruation is the way a girl's body gets ready for having a baby some day. It's a normal, natural and healthy thing and usually doesn't hurt, even though the drips might look like blood.

*In the next section...*

*You might be wondering What kinds of questions can I expect my child to ask at this age? Or, What are the things other parents want to know? We asked our experts and they put together some of the most popular questions children and parents ask along with the answers.*

# 25 Quick Answers to Tough Questions

We've sourced some of the toughest questions kids and parents ask… and we've provided answers!

## 17 Quick Answers for Kids:

### 1. How does a baby get in mommy's tummy?

*Why do you ask? What do you think? Babies are made when an egg from a woman's body joins with a sperm from a man's body.*

### 2. How are babies born?

*Great question! What's your guess? A baby usually comes out of an opening between a woman's legs called the vagina but sometimes a doctor does an operation to get the baby out.*

### 3. Did you and dad do that?

*Simple answer: yes or no!*

### 4. How did you get me?

*Insert appropriate answer, being as honest (and scientific) as possible!*

### 5. How are babies made?

*There are lots of different ways that babies are made. Usually when a man and a woman want to make a baby, the man puts his penis inside the woman's vagina to join the sperm and the egg.*

### 6. Why don't boys have boobs?

*Boys do have breasts. They're just smaller because they don't have to carry milk.*

### 7. Why don't I have a penis/vagina?

*A boy is usually born with a penis and a girl is usually born with a vagina.*

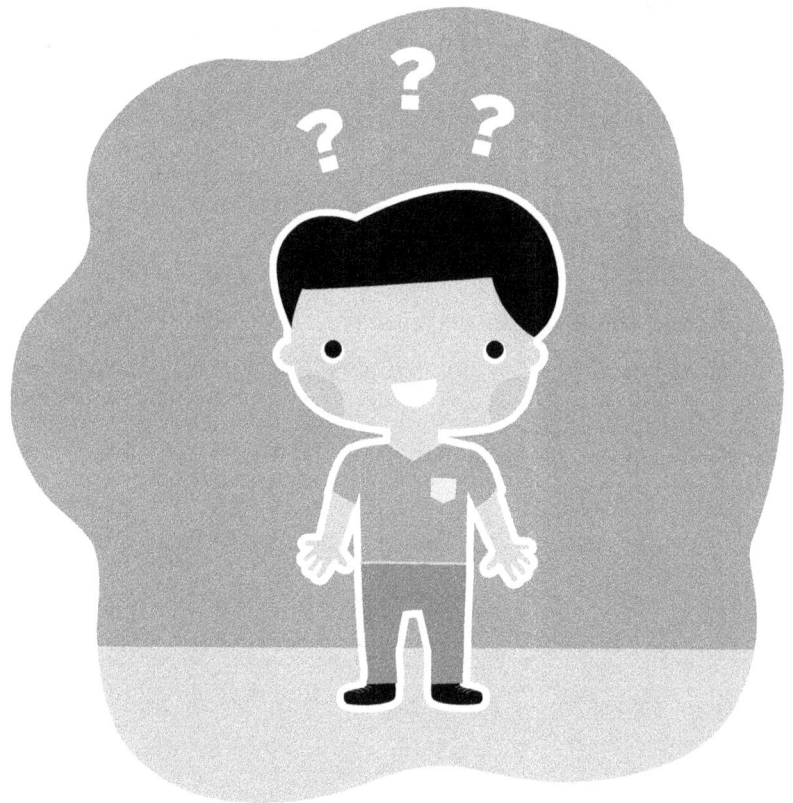

46

**8. What happened to my penis?**

*You never had a penis because you're a girl.*

**9. Why does Paul stand up to pee, and I have to sit?**

*Urine comes out of an opening called the urethra. Boys have longer urethras than girls so they can stand to urinate.*

**10. Can I see where the baby came out of you?**

*The baby came out of my vagina but it's a part of my body that I keep private.*

**11. Why do you have hair down there?**

*Nice observation! Why do you think? Hair on the genitals is called pubic hair and it keeps that area clean.*

**12. Can I practice kissing you?**

*No, I'm not comfortable with that because romantic kissing is not something that parents and their children do.*

**13. Why does my vagina tickle?**

*That feeling is normal and healthy. It means that your body is working properly. But let's remember that those feelings are private.*

**14. My Penis is magic. It goes up and down when I touch it.**

*It's not magic. The flow of blood inside makes the penis go up and down. Boys have these practice erections several times a day. It's a healthy sign that they're getting ready to have babies someday.*

**15. Can I have a baby when I get big?**

*Sure! When you're an adult you can make that decision.*

**16. Can I marry you Mommy/Daddy?**

*No, kids can't marry their parents. But I will be your mommy/daddy forever!*

**17. Can I marry my sister?**

*No, it's against the law to marry a family member.*

# 8 Quick Answers for Parents:

**1. Our son walked in on us having sex and I'm not sure how to handle it.**

*Politely ask your son to leave the room, letting him know that you'll be with him momentarily. When talking to him, explain that you and his mom/dad/your partner were having some private time together. Often, children are concerned that someone is being hurt so assure your son that this isn't the case, reminding him that adults engage in these activities to show their love and affection for one another.*

**2. My daughter saw inappropriate sexual content on the Internet. What should I do?**

*Explain that some images on the Internet are meant for adults only. Praise your daughter for telling you about it and encourage her to do the same in the future. Depending on the nature of the content, stress that what she saw wasn't real.*

**3. How much do I tell my child about how babies are created?**

*Everything! Provide small increments of information, answer questions as they arise, and let them show you when their curiosity has been satisfied.*

**4. What is age appropriate?**

*Any adult topic that relates to emotional, physical and sexual health. If the information you provide your child is irrelevant or premature, they won't retain it.*

**5. Won't telling my daughter about sex early only heighten her curiosity and encourage her to become sexual younger?**

*Actually, research shows that children who are taught about sex early tend to delay sexual activity. It's ignorance and curiosity (not knowledge) that leads to earlier sexual experimentation.*

**6. If I sexually inform my son, won't it encourage him want to act it out in play?**

*No. Not if you teach him that sex is only for adults and that it's not okay for children to act it out, even if they are just playing.*

**7. I'm uncomfortable with the interest my daughter has taken in my body. Is her behaviour normal?**

*Yes, it's very normal. If your child asks you to touch their genitals, or to touch or look at yours, don't be afraid to express your boundaries.*

**8. I've always had pet names for my private parts. Is there anything really wrong with using this language with my child?**

*Studies show that children who are informed and comfortable with their bodies are more protected from abuse. Using the right words for your privates shows your child that you're not ashamed of your body and you're open to future conversations. Knowledge is protection.*

---

We hope you've enjoyed your journey through **Sex Education: It's More Than Learning About How Babies Are Made!** for parents with Preschool children. We welcome your feedback and would love to know what you think. Please take the time to rate us, leave a comment or contact us directly at: mail@birdeesapp.com.

*If you're wondering what's in store for you as your child enters the Primary School years, we've outlined what you can expect next...*

# WHAT TO EXPECT NEXT

Parenting becomes more challenging as children's perceptions begin evolving with new perspectives predicated on rules, logic, and facts.

Here's what you can expect from children ages 6-8:

## Independence

- *preferring to socialize with their own gender*
- *referencing external sources for answer to questions*
- *touching their genitals for pleasure or comfort*
- *same-gender sexual exploration*
- *body proprietorship manifesting as shyness and modesty*
- *owning the right to say NO*

What do children ages 6-8 need?

## Context

- *sexual dialogue is important*
- *facts should not be confused with knowledge*
- *knowledge ensures health, respect, and safety in future relationships*
- *knowledge makes targeting by predators less likely*
- *sex is more than reproduction*
- *boundaries exist and should be respected*
- *bodies are private and should be respected*
- *understanding puberty*
- *understanding diversity*
- *understanding gender role stereotypes*

**Sex Education: Curiosity Is Getting Complicated!** Outlines the information that you should convey to your child as they grow through the ages of 6 to 8. It includes strategies for answering questions, and resources to assist their implementation. **Sex Education: Curiosity Is Getting Complicated!** Is available for purchase at: **www.birdeesapp.com**

# WHAT DOES THAT MEAN?

**Anus**: the opening at the end of our digestive tract (between our buttocks) where stool/solid waste exits the body

**Breasts**: glandular organs situated on the upper chest that are more developed in woman and are used to secrete milk after childbirth to feed the newborn baby

**Circumcision**: the surgical removal of the foreskin (fold of skin) that covers the tip of the penis

**Clitoris**: a tiny knob about as big as the end of a little finger that sits above the vulva (labia)

**Condom**: a thin sheath usually made of rubber that is worn on the penis in men and in the vagina in woman that acts as a barrier to prevent unwanted pregnancies or to provide protection from sexually transmitted infections

**Empathy**: being able to understand what someone else may be thinking, feeling or experiencing

**Erection(s)**: when a penis becomes hard and stands away from the body, due to a rush of blood into its spongy tissue

**Foreskin**: a retractable fold of skin that covers the glans(tip) of the penis

**Fraternal Twins**: twins that are made when two eggs are fertilized by two sperm at the same time

**Gay**: a term used to describe a homosexual man or woman

**Gender**: a person's own sense of being either male or female

**Gender Identity**: a person's own view of being male, female, both or neither

**Gender Variant**: a person that doesn't conform to being male or female

**Genitals**: internal and external male and female sex organs involved in reproduction

**Heterosexual**: someone that is physically/sexually attracted to members of the opposite sex

**Homosexual**: someone that is physically/sexually attracted to members of the same sex

**Lesbian**: a woman that is physically/sexually attracted to other women

**Masturbation**: touching one's own body and genitals for sexual pleasure

**Menarche**: the first menstrual bleeding that a female experiences

**Menstruation/Period**: monthly shedding of the lining of the uterus that moves out of the uterus through the cervix and comes out of the vagina as menstrual blood drops that lasts from 3-5 days

**Ovary(ies)**: the female sex organs that produce ova(um) (eggs)

**Penis**: the part of the external male sex organ that is designed to deliver sperm into the vagina

**Pregnant**: carrying a developing baby inside the womb

**Private**: belonging to that person and not intended for public display or other people

**Privates or Private Parts**: the genitals, breasts, and mouth

**Puberty**: the period in a young person's life (age 8-18) when their child body gradually changes into an adult body

**Queer**: a man who is physically/sexually attracted to other men

**Scrotum**: an elastic protective pouch of skin that surrounds the testicles.

**Sex**: a way to describe whether a person is of male or female based on their external genitals

**Sex/Intercourse**: the act of the penis penetrating the vagina, or any consensual behaviour between two or more individuals of the same or opposite sex involving genital contact and bodily penetration

**Sex Organs**: the parts of the body that are involved in reproduction and that distinguish us as being male or female based on those organs

**Sexual**: relating to sex

**Sexual Deviancy**: abnormal sexual behaviour

**Sexual Diversity**: issues relating to sexual orientation and gender identity

**Sexual Orientation**: the emotional, romantic or physical attraction to people of the same, opposite, both, or neither gender

**Sexuality**: the way people express themselves as sexual beings or the awareness of being either males or female or the way someone is physically attracted to other people

**Shame(ful)**: the feeling that you've done something wrong that needs to be covered up or hidden away from others

**Smegma**: a secretion (white cheesy substance) from the genitals that collects between the labial folds in females and foreskin of males

**Sperm**: the male seed or reproductive cell

**Stool**: the solid waste produced by the digestive system

**Testicles (Testes)**: male sex organs that produce sperm/seed

**Testosterone**: a male hormone produced by the testicles, that is responsible for growth and sexual development

**Transgendered**: an individual who identifies with or relates to a gender different to the one that was present at birth

**Transsexual**: an individual who identifies psychologically with a gender opposite to that of their assigned sex at birth to the point that they want to surgically change their sex

**Twins**: two babies that are conceived and born at the same time

**Urethra**: the tube that carries urine from the bladder out of the body through the penis in men and the urethral opening in women

**Urine**: liquid waste produced by the urinary system that comes out of the body through the urethra

**Uterus** (Womb): a muscular sac-like organ that houses the developing fetus until birth

**Vagina**: a tube-like passageway connecting the labia (external genitalia) to the uterus (womb), which acts as a sheath for the penis during intercourse and expands to allow the baby to pass through it during childbirth

**Vulva (Labia)**: the inner (minora) and outer (majora) folds of skin surrounding the vaginal opening

# SOURCES AND RESOURCES

## Websites

www.advocatesforyouth.org

www.ashastd.org

www.betterhealth.vic.gov.au

www.birdeesapp.com

www.cfsh.ca

www.crossmap.christianpost.com

www.familieslikemine.com

www.genderspectrum.org

www.goaskalice.columbia.ed

www.guttmacher.org

www.imatyfa.org

www.iwannaknow.org

www.kidshealth.org

www.oprah.com

www.optionsforsexualhealth.org

www.pflag.org

www.pflagcanada.ca

www.planetahead.ca

www.plannedparenthood.org

www.teachingsexualhealth.ca

www.safehealthschools.org

www.sexetc.org

www.sexualityandu.ca

www.sieccan.org

www.siecus.org

www.transactiveonline.org

www.urbandictionary.com

# Adult Books

Berman, Dr. Laura. *The Sex Ed Handbook: A Comprehensive Guide for Parents.* Nov. 2012. http://Oprah.com2011

Berkenkamp, Laurie and Steven Atkins. *Talking to your Kids about Sex: A Go Parents! Guide.* Norwich, VT: Nomad Press, 2002.

Brill, Stephanie and Rachel Pepper. *The Transgender Child: A Handbook for Families and Professionals.* San Francisco, CA: Cleis Press Inc, 2008.

Faber, Adele and Elaine Mazlish. *How to Talk So Kids Will Listen & Listen So Kids will Talk.* Updated ed. New York, NY: Scribner, 2012.

Regional Municipality of Halton. Children and Sexuality: *A Guide for Parents and Caregivers of young Children.* www.halton.ca/common/pages/UserFile.aspx?fileId=15448> Halton Region, 2012

Heyman, Richard. *We Need to Talk! Tough Conversations with your Kids: From Sex to Family Values, Tackle Any Topic with Sensitivity and Smarts.* Avon, MA: Adams Media, 2009.

Hickling, Meg. *Boys, Girls and Body Science: A first Book about Facts of Life.* Madeira Park, BC: Harbour Publishing Co. Ltd., 2002.

Hickling, Meg. *The New Speaking of Sex: What Your Children Need to Know and When They Need to Know it.* Kelowna, BC: Northstone, 2005.

Kaeser, Dr. Fred. *What Your Child Needs to Know About Sex (and When): A Straight Talking Guide For Parents.* New York, NY: Celestial Arts, 2011.

Levine, Judith. Harmful to Minors: *The Perils of Protecting Children from Sex.* Minneapolis, MN: University of Minnesota Press, 2002.

Maxwell, Sharon. *The Talk: What Your Kids Need to Hear From YOU About Sex.* Penguin Group

(USA) Inc., New York, NY: 2008

Public Health Agency of Canada. *Canadian Guidelines for Sexual Health Education, 2008*. Ottawa, ON: Published by Authority of the Minister of Health, 2008

Public Health Agency of Canada, Minister of Health. *Questions & Answers: Sexual Orientation in Schools*. Published by Authority of the Minister of Health <library.catie.ca/pdf/ATI-20000s/26288E.pdf>.

Rebecca White. *Sex and Relationship Education in Primary School: Professional Development File*. Optimus Professional Publishing Ltd, 2010.

Roffman, Deborah M. *Sex and Sensibility: The Thinking Parent's Guide to Talking Sense About Sex*. Cambridge, MA: Perseus, 2001.

Rosenzweig, Janet.*The Sex-Wise Parent: The Parent's Guide to Protecting Your Child, Strengthening Your Family, and Talking to Kids about Sex, Abuse and Bullying*. New York, NY: Skyhorse Publishing Inc., 2012.

St. Stephen's Community House. *The Little Black Book for Girlz: A Book on Healthy Sexuality*. Toronto, ON: Annick press Ltd., 2008.

St. Stephen's Community House - By Youth for Youth. *The Little Black Book for Guys: Guys Talk About Sex*. Toronto, ON: Annick Press Ltd., 2010.

Sexuality Information and Education Council of the United States. *Guidelines for Comprehensive Sexuality Education: Kindergarten through 12th Grade 3rd ed*. National Guidelines Task Force, 2004. <www2.gsu.edu/guidelines.pdf>

Schwartz, Pepper. *Ten Talks Parents Must Have With Their Children About Sex and Character*. New York, NY: Hyperion, 2000.

Wass, Patricia C. *Summer Time - Sex Education Helps Keep Children Safe from Abuse*. <http://crossmap.christianpost.com/news/summer-time-sex-education-helps-keep-children-safe-from-abuse-3195> Crossmap, June 2013.

# Children's Books

Bourgeois, Paulette and Kim Martyn. *Changes in You and Me: A Book About Puberty, Mostly for Girls, rev ed.* Toronto, ON: Key Porter Books, 2005.

Bourgeois, Paulette & Kim Martyn. *Changes in You and Me: A Book About Puberty, Mostly for Boys, rev ed.* Toronto, ON: Key Porter Books, 2005.

Carr, Jennifer. *Be Who You Are.* Bloomington, IN: Authorhouse, 2010.

Carlson, Nancy. *My family is Forever.* New York: Viking Books, 2004.

Cole, Joanna. *Asking About Sex and Growing Up: A Question-and-Answer Book for Kids.* New York, NY: Harpers Collins, 2009.

Firth, Alex. *What's Happening to Me?* (Boys Edition). London, UK: Usborne Publishing Ltd., 2006.

Harris, Robie H. It's Perfectly Normal: *Changing Bodies, Growing Up, Sex, and Sexual Health.* Cambridge, MA: Candlewick Press, 2009.

Harris, Robie H. *It's so Amazing!: A Book about Eggs, Sperm, Birth, Babies and Families.* Cambridge, MA: Candlewick Press, 2004.

Harris, Robie H. *It's Not the Stork!: A Book about Girls, Boys, Babies, Bodies, Families and Friends.* Cambridge, MA: Candlewick Press, 2008.

Hickling, Meg. *Boys, Girls and Body Science: A first Book about Facts of Life.* Madeira Park, BC: Harbour Publishing Co. Ltd., 2002

Hindman, Jan. A very Touching Book. Ontario, OR: Alexandria Assoc, 1990.

King, Zack and Kimberly King. *I Said No! A Kid-to-Kid Guide to Keeping Private Parts Private.* Weaverville, CA: Boulden, 2010.

Mayle, Peter. *Where did I Come From?* New York, NY: Kensington - Citadel, 1977.

Mayle, Peter. *What's Happening to Me?* New York, NY: Kensington - Citadel, 1981.

Meredith, Susan. *What's happening to me?* (Girls Edition). London, UK: Usborne Publishing Ltd., 2006.

Stones, Rosemary. *Where Do BabiesCome From?* New York, NY: Puffin Books, 1989